The Pharmacy Doesn't Have the Cure to Diseases; it's in Nature

ChrisAngela Spencer

WE Shine Media Solutions

Publishing Company: WE Shine Media Solutions

ISBN 978-1-304-11920-9

Printed in: The United States, First Edition

Disclaimer

The information presented in this book is for educational purposes only and is not intended as a substitute for professional medical advice, diagnosis, or treatment. While herbal remedies have been traditionally used in various cultures for health and wellness, their effectiveness and safety may vary depending on the individual, the condition being treated, and other factors.

Please Note:

- Always consult with a qualified healthcare professional before beginning any new treatment, including herbal remedies.
- The herbal remedies discussed in this book have not been evaluated by the Food and Drug Administration (FDA) or any other regulatory body for the treatment, cure, or prevention of any disease.
- Individual results may vary. The use of herbs and supplements should be based on your own research and in consultation with your healthcare provider.
- Some herbs may interact with prescription medications or other treatments, and may not be suitable for all individuals, including pregnant or nursing women, children, or those with pre-existing health conditions.
- The author and publisher of this book disclaim any liability for any adverse effects, consequences, or damages resulting from the use or misuse of the information contained herein.

By reading this book, you acknowledge that the author and publisher are not responsible for any outcomes related to the use of herbal remedies or other information provided in this text.

The Pharmacy Doesn't Have the Cure to Diseases; it's in Nature

"Heal naturally from what the earth yields. For every disease, there's a natural remedy to cure you."

~ChrisAngela Spencer~

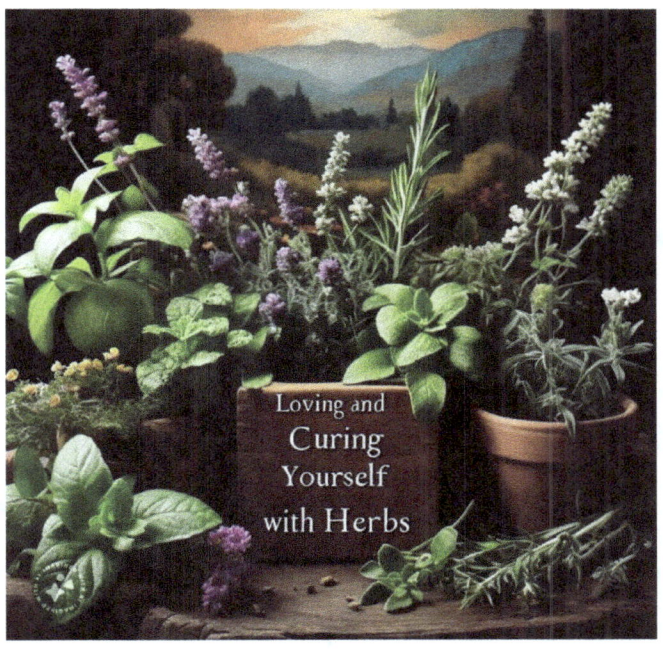

Changing your diet is a powerful tool in managing your health. It requires real discipline, but it's worth it. The herbs you consume drive out mucus, cancers, parasites, and metal calcifications from your body, and then these toxins are eliminated through urination or defecation. Trust the process, trust the herbs, and remember to drink plenty of fluids to aid in the detoxification process.

~ChrisAngela Spencer~

Table of Contents

Chapter 1

Hypertension -HBP (High Blood Pressure)

High blood pressure is a condition in which the force of the blood against the artery walls is too high, which may be caused by a lack of physical activity and too much salt in the diet. Plaque buildup in the arteries, called atherosclerosis, increases the risk of high blood pressure.

Stage 1 high blood pressure, also known as hypertension, is a blood pressure reading of 130–139 mmHg systolic or 80–89 mmHg diastolic. Stage 2 high blood pressure is considered 140/90 or higher. It is considered extremely high if your blood pressure reading is 180/120 or higher. So, you have to be very cautious and seek help.

Deep breathing for 15-20 minutes can lower blood pressure. Slow, deep breathing relaxes and dilates the blood vessels. It can also stimulate the lymphatic system, which helps to detoxify the body.

Sipping tea is another way to help manage blood pressure naturally. This herbal blend assists with fighting high blood pressure and stabilizes the immune and digestive systems.

High Blood Pressure Tea

1. Hawthorn
2. Angelica root
3. Hibiscus
4. Elderberry
5. Yarrow

HAWTHORN

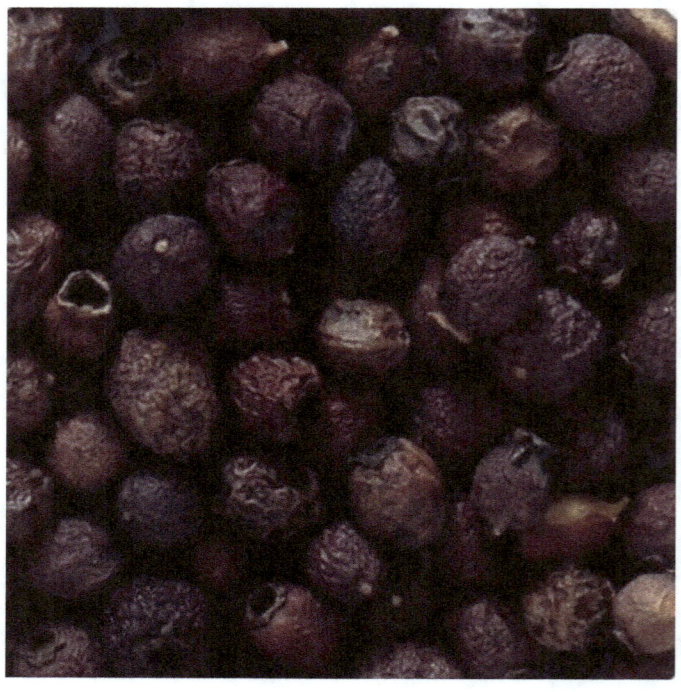

Crataegus, commonly called hawthorn, grows in temperate regions throughout the world. Historically, hawthorn has been used for heart disease as well as for digestive and kidney problems. It is now promoted for these uses as well as for anxiety, high or low blood pressure, and other conditions. (https://en.wikipedia.org/wiki/Crataegus)

ANGELICA ROOT

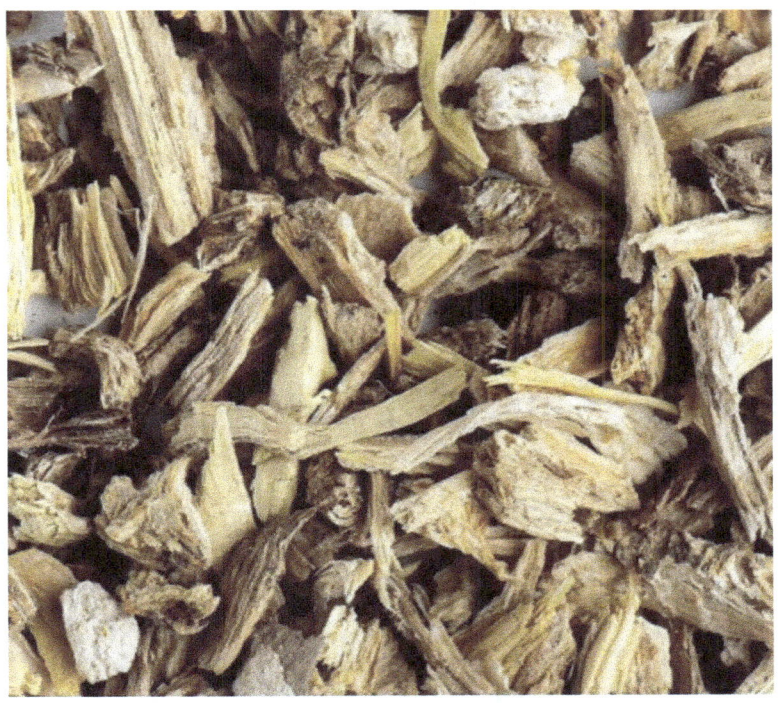

Angelica Root, also known as dong quai (Angelica sinensis), is a plant used in Chinese medicine to treat hypertension.

(https://www.healthline.com/nutrition/angelica-root).

HIBISCUS

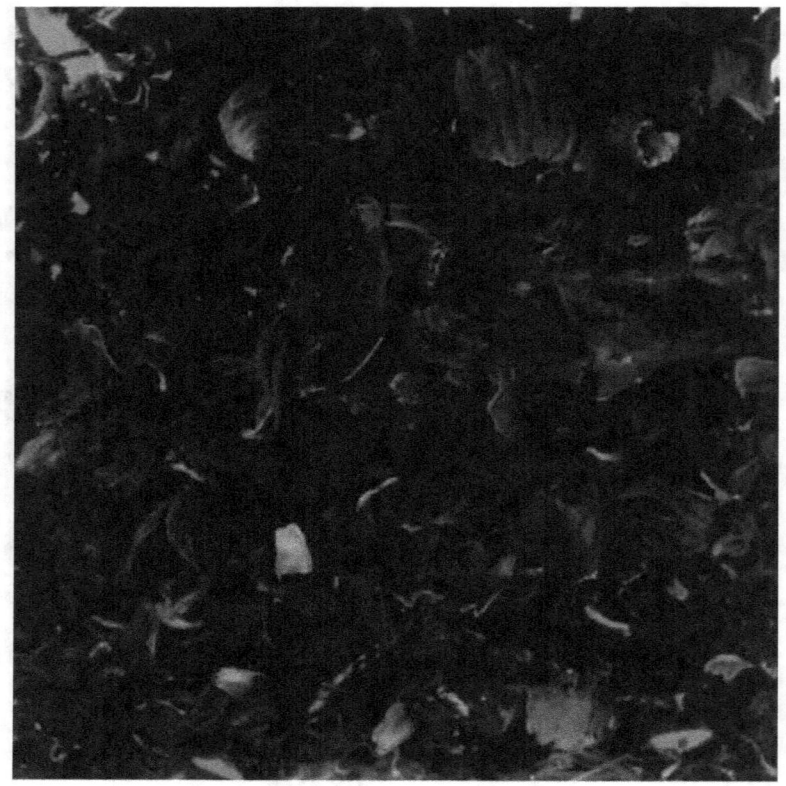

Hibiscus is a genus of flowering plants in the mallow family, Malvaceae. Hibiscus preparations, including teas, powders, and extracts, have been shown to decrease blood pressure, reduce body fat, improve metabolic syndrome, protect the liver, and fight cancer cells.
(https://www.healthline.com/health/all-you-need-to -know-hibiscus).

ELDERBERRY

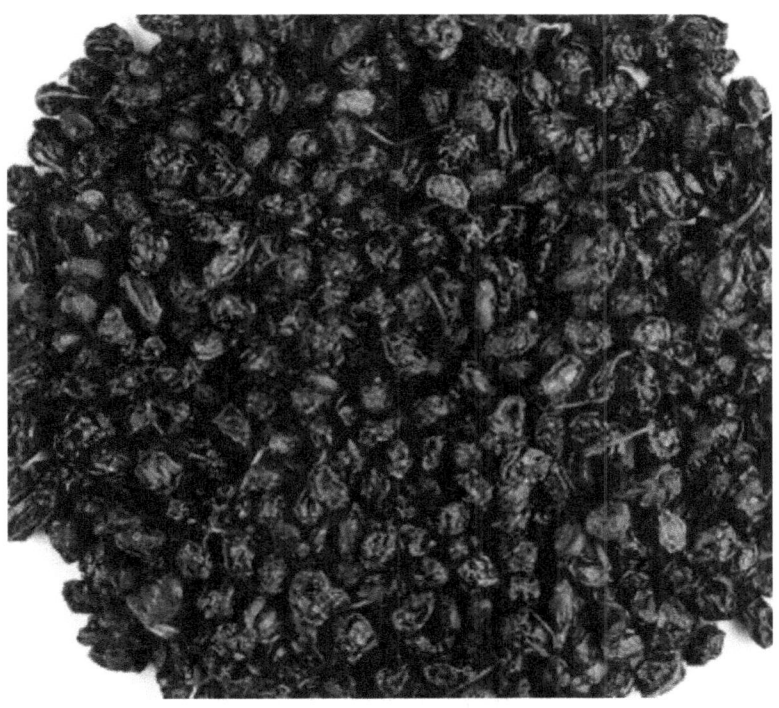

Elderberry is the dark purple berry of the
European or black elder tree, which grows in
the warmer parts of Europe, North America,
Asia, and Northern Africa. It is rich in
antioxidants, which can help lower
inflammation as well as cholesterol and
blood pressure.
(https://www.health.com/health-benefits-of-
elderberry-7506026).

YARROW

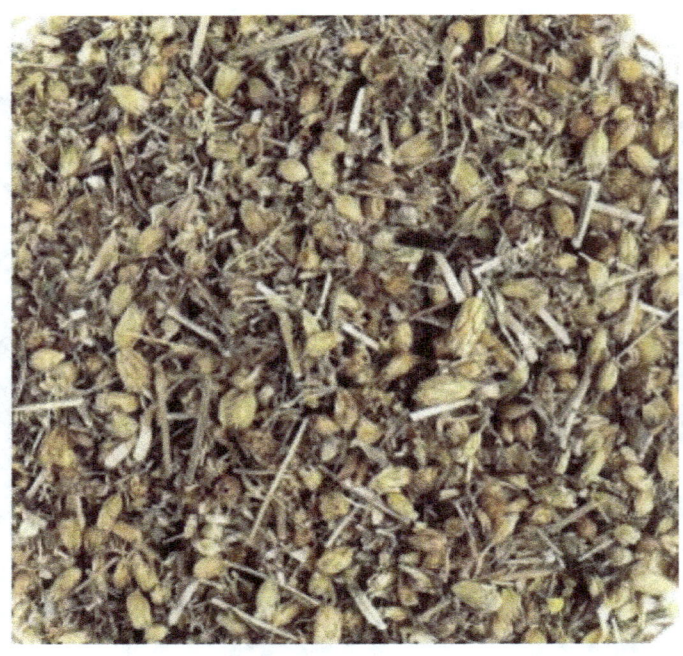

Yarrow - Achillea millefolium, commonly known as yarrow or common yarrow, is a flowering plant in the family Asteraceae. Yarrow may lower blood pressure slightly and could strengthen the effects of prescription drugs taken to lower blood pressure.
(https://www.mountsinai.org/health-library/herb/yarrow).

Chapter 2

Thyroids

The thyroid is a small butterfly-shaped gland in the front of your neck. It makes hormones that control the way the body uses energy. These hormones affect nearly every organ in your body and control many of your body's most important functions. Problems with the thyroid can be caused by iodine deficiency.

Thyroid tea helps to regulate normal thyroid activity. This blend offers a nourishing blend of six herbs to support optimal thyroid function and overall well-being. Consume 2-3 glasses daily.

Thyroid Tea

1. Ashwagandha Root

2. Ginger Root

3. Gotu Kola

4. Holy Basil

5. Lemon Balm

6. Nettle

ASHWAGANDHA ROOT

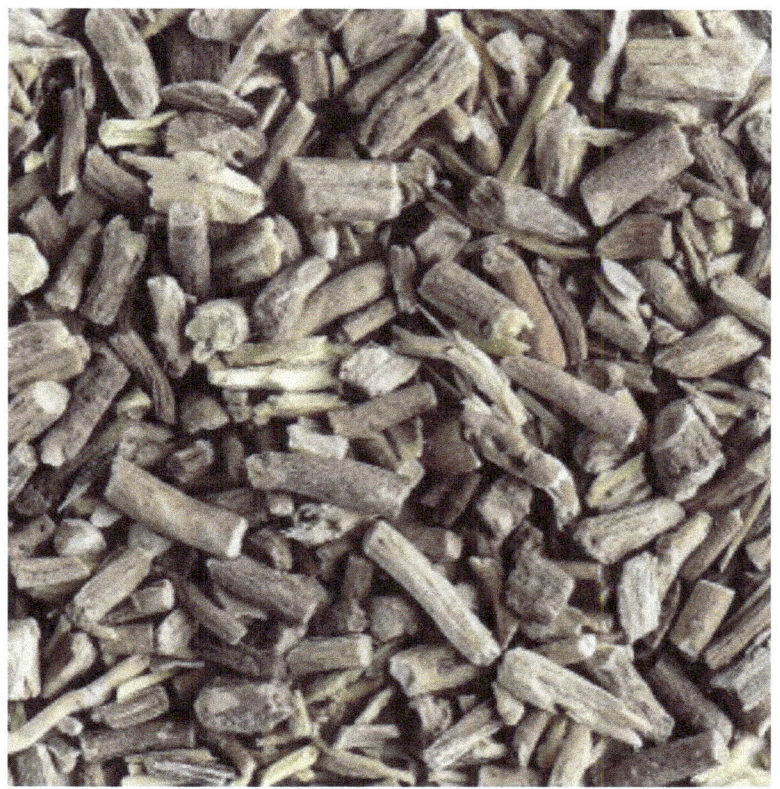

Ashwagandha root is an evergreen shrub that grows in Asia and Africa. Studies have found that ashwagandha can lead to significant improvements in thyroid levels. (https://www.medicalnewstoday.com/articles/ashwagandha-and-thyroid)

GINGER ROOT

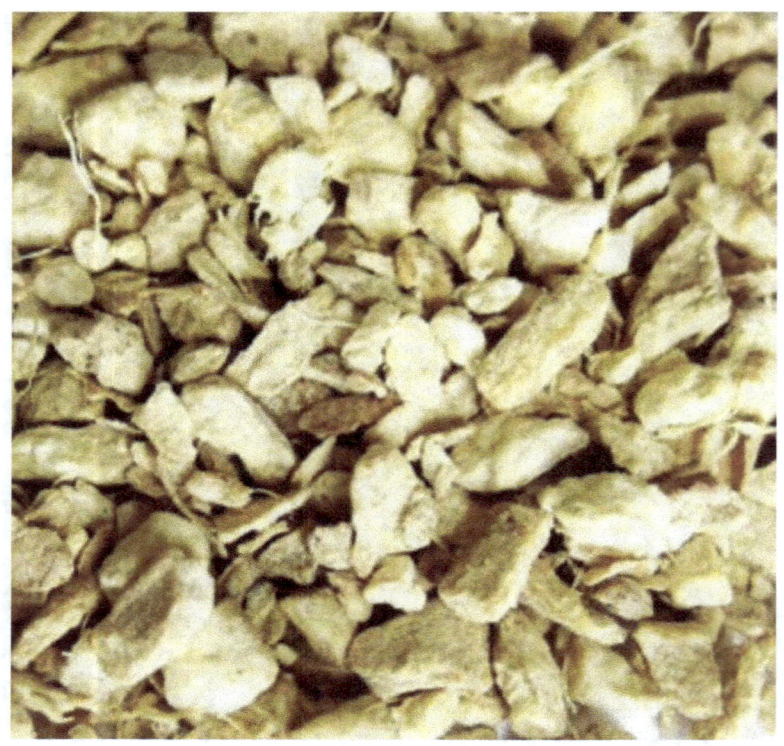

Ginger root is rich in essential minerals like potassium and magnesium and helps combat inflammation, one of the primary causes of thyroid issues.
(https://pharmeasy.in/blog/11-home-remedies-for-thyroid/)

GOTU KOLA

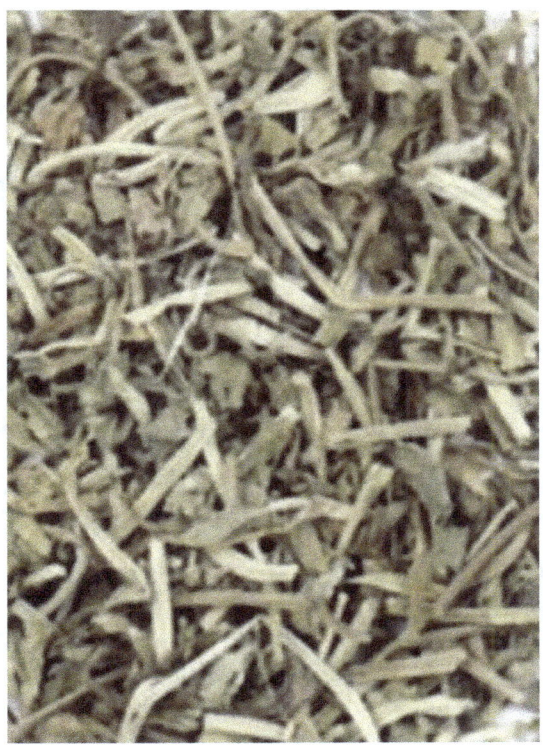

Gotu kola (Centella Asiatica) is an herb in the parsley family. It has a long history of use in the traditional Chinese and Ayurvedic medicine systems. Gotu kola, another adaptogenic herb, is believed to support thyroid function by stimulating the production of thyroid hormones.
(https://americanherbalistsguild.com/sites/default/files/sinadinos_christa_-_herbal_support_for_hypothyroidism.pdf)

HOLY BASIL

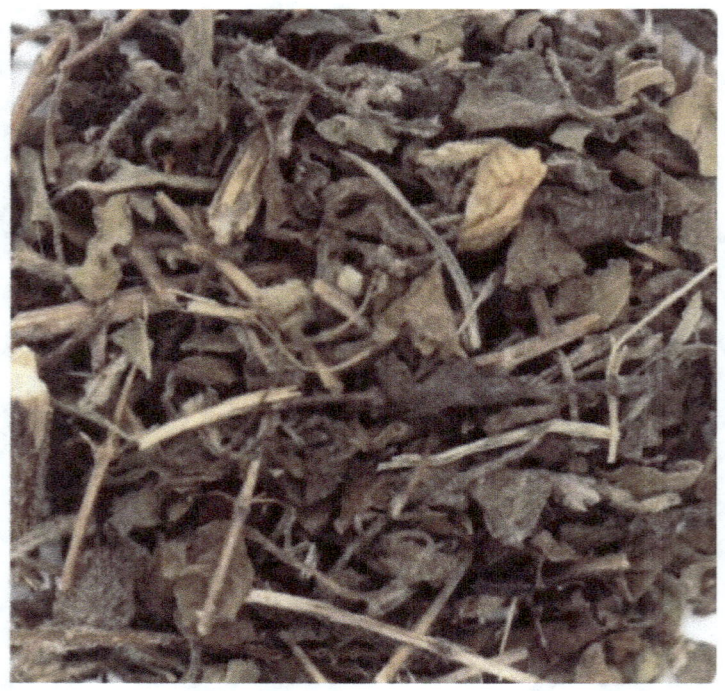

Holy basil (Ocimum tenuiflorum) is a plant that is native to India. It is commonly used in the traditional Indian medicine system, Ayurveda. Using holy basil may improve your thyroid health by balancing the cortisol levels first.

(https://www.mindbodygreen.com/articles/the-side-effects-of-holy-basil-you-may-not-know-about-seo)

LEMON BALM

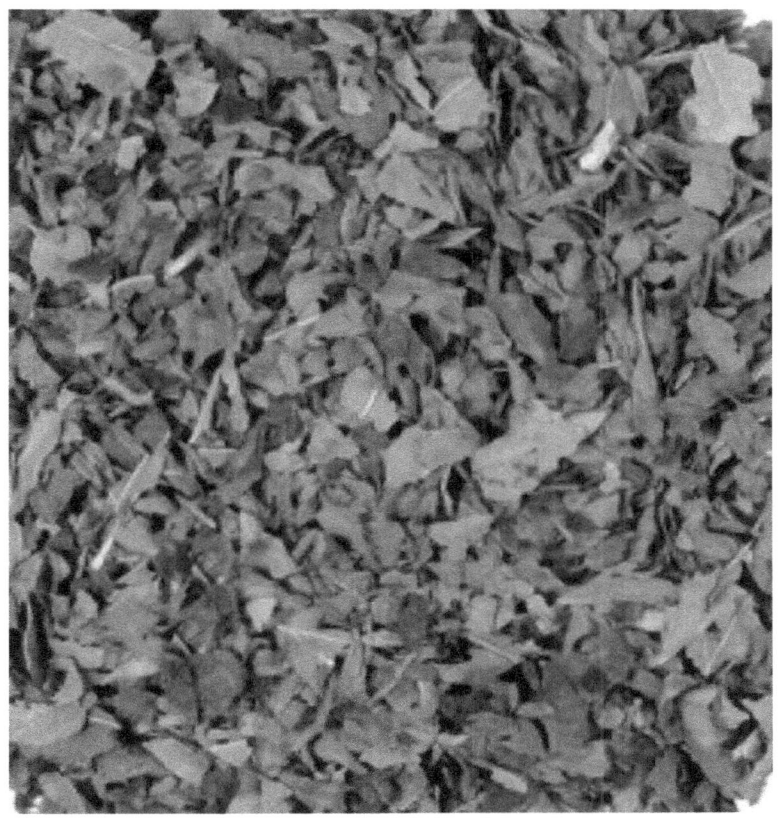

Lemon balm (Melissa officinalis) is an herb from the mint family. This low-growing, herbaceous plant has been used traditionally for mood disorders, insomnia, infections, and the symptoms of hyperthyroidism.
(https://restorativemedicine.org/library/monographs/lemon-balm-melissa-officinalis-2/)

NETTLE

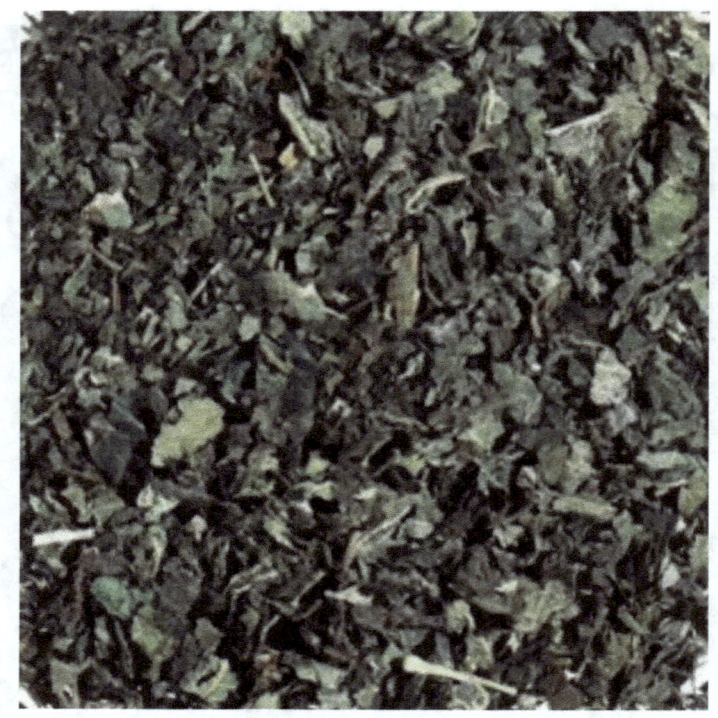

Nettle, a nutrient-dense herb, is rich in vitamins and minerals that are essential for thyroid health. Nettle also contains A and B Vitamins. Vitamin A has been linked to regulating thyroid hormone metabolism. (https://nutratea.co.uk/blogs/supplements-for -thyroid-health/)

Chapter 3

Fibroids (Uterine Myoma)

Fibroids are noncancerous growths in the uterus that can develop during the childbearing years of a woman's life. Fibroids include heavy menstrual bleeding, prolonged periods, and in some cases pelvic pain.

This herbal tea blend can shrink the growth of fibroids by bringing down inflammation and high estrogen levels. It may also improve symptoms of heavy bleeding due to fibroids. Consume 2-3 glasses daily.

Fibroid Tea

1. Burdock Root

2. Ginger

3. Turmeric

4. Dandelion Root

5. Chaste tree berries

BURDOCK ROOT

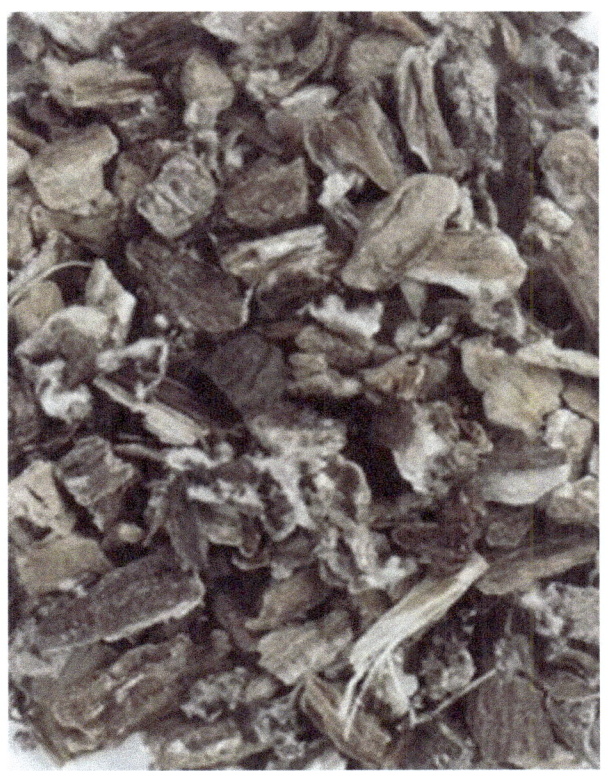

Burdock root (Arctium lappa) is a plant native to Japan that is now found all over the world. Burdock root is a good source of antioxidants, which are chemical compounds that help protect your cells from damage.

(https://www.ncbi.nlm.nih.gov/pmc/articles/PMC7 478476/)

GINGER

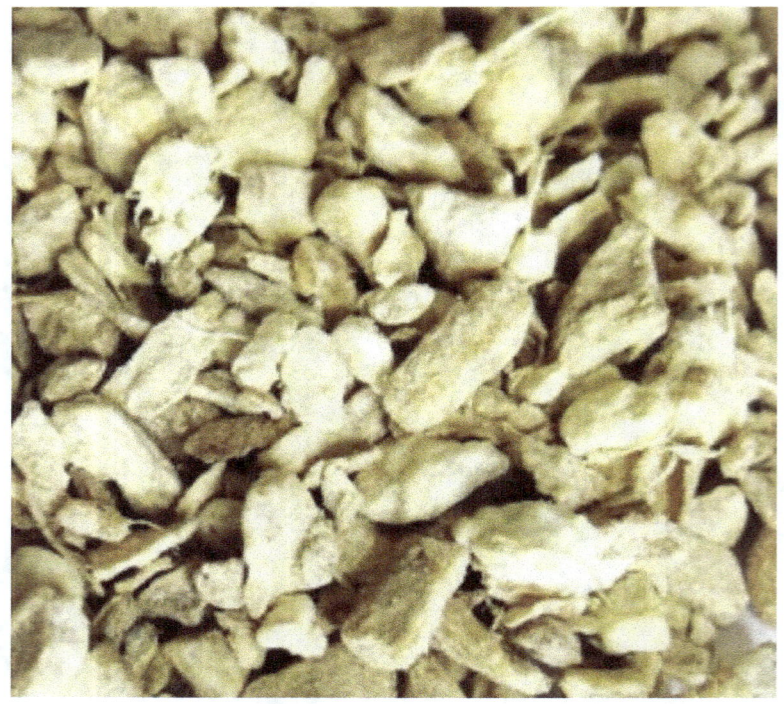

Ginger (Zingiber officinale) is a plant native to Asia. The ginger spice comes from the roots of the plant. It's used as a food flavoring and medicine. One of the most popular natural remedies that is usually recommended to shrink fibroids is ginger.

(https://fibroidnaturalhealing.quora.com/Can -Ginger-Shrink-Uterine-Fibroids)

TURMERIC

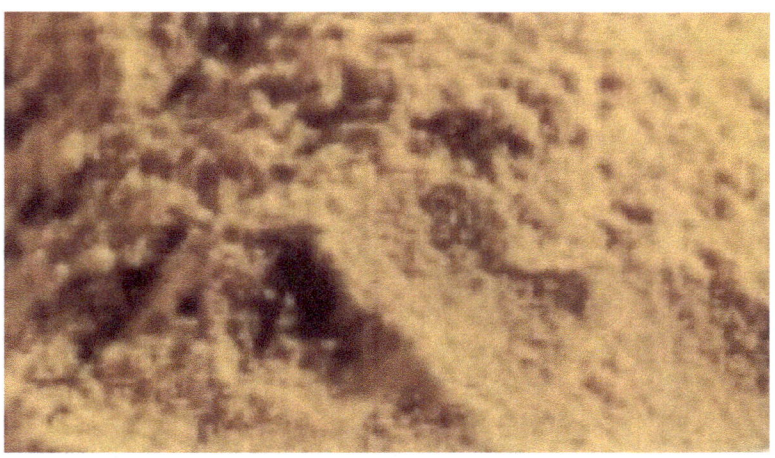

Turmeric is a deep, golden-orange spice known for adding color, flavor, and nutrition to foods. Some research suggests that turmeric may help with uterine fibroids.

Turmeric contains curcumin, an antioxidant and anti-inflammatory that may inhibit fibroid growth and destroy or stop fibroid cells from reproducing. (https://www.ncbi.nlm.nih.gov/pmc/articles/PMC9256340/)

DANDELION

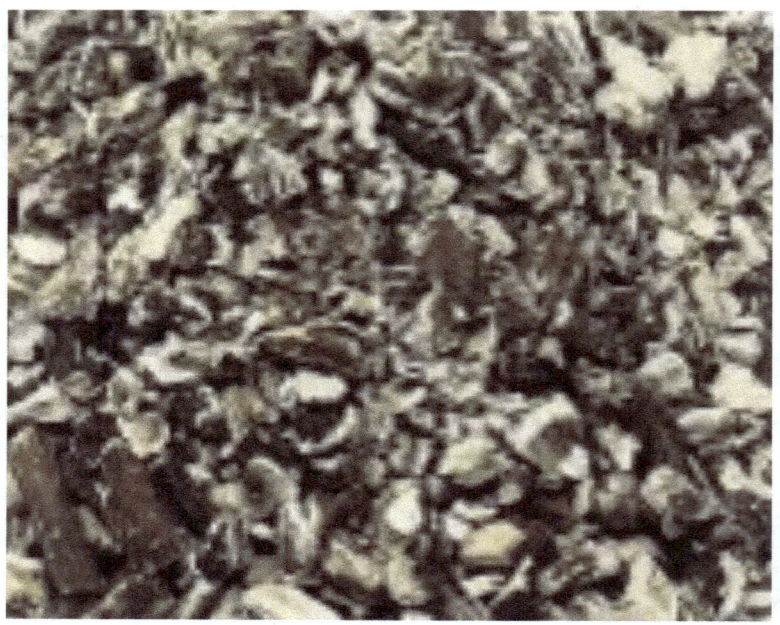

Dandelion is native to Europe but found throughout temperate regions in the Northern Hemisphere. The leaves, flowers, and root of the plant have traditionally been used in Mexican and other North American medicine. Today, dandelion is promoted as a "tonic," as a diuretic, and for a variety of conditions. (https://www.healthline.com/health/ways-dandelion-tea-could-be-good-for-your)

CHASTE TREE BERRIES

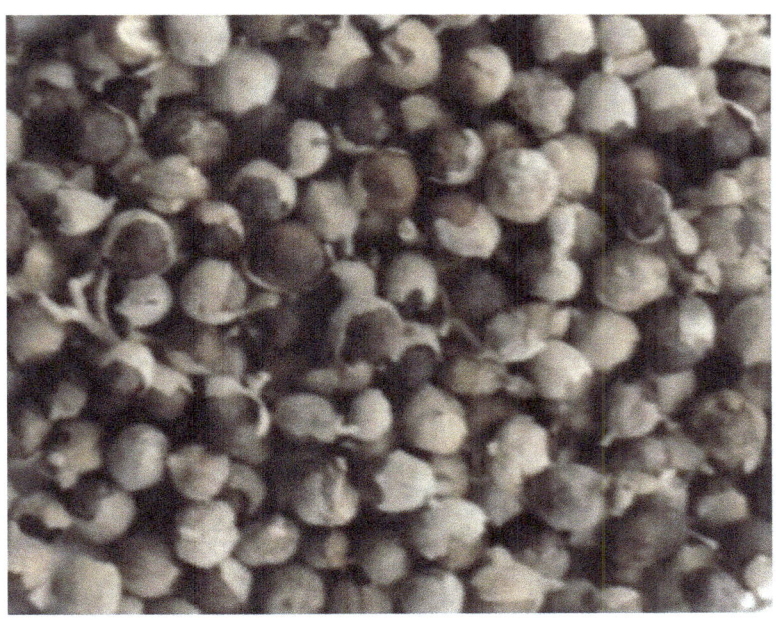

Chaste tree berries are also known as vitex or monk's pepper. A key way to prevent and reduce uterine fibroids is to maintain a proper balance of hormones. Chasteberry can help to balance the ratio of estrogen to progesterone. (https://draxe.com/nutrition/vitex/#:~:text=R educes%20Uterine%20Fibroids&text=A%2 0key%20way%20to%20prevent,ratio%20of %20estrogen%20to%20progesterone.)

Chapter 4

Kidney Stones (Nephrolithiasis)

Kidney stones are hard deposits of minerals and acid salts that stick together in concentrated urine. They can be painful when passing through the urinary tract but usually don't cause permanent damage. Kidney stones pass through the ureter and bladder.

This tea blend aids in the passing of kidney stones and supports the treatment of the kidneys after passing the stones. It has beneficial therapeutic effects on the urinary tract and kidney stones. Consume 2-3 glasses daily.

Kidney Stone Tea

1. Burdock Root

2. Horsetail

3. Rosemary

4. Stinging Nettle Leaf

5. Goldenrod

BURDOCK ROOT

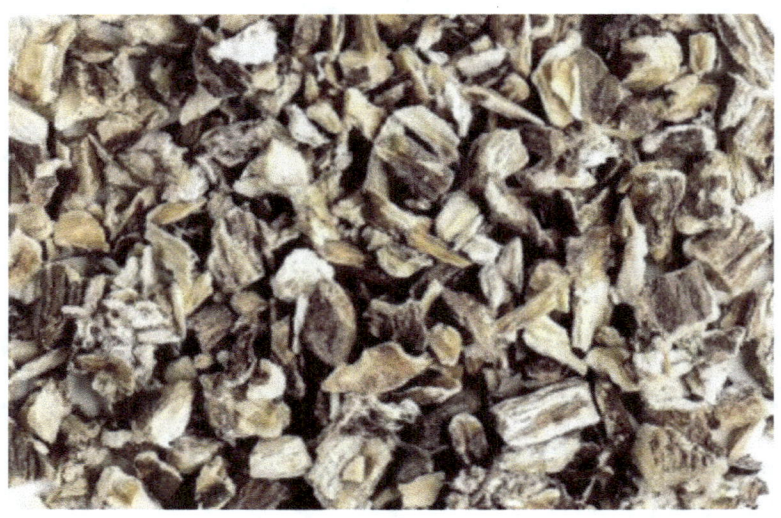

Burdock root acts as a natural blood and lymphatic cleanser. It helps your body remove toxins from your blood through your lymphatic system before being filtered by your kidneys. Essentially, it helps your kidneys function more efficiently. (https://humantonik.com/burdock-root-benefits/#:~:text=or%20kidney%20failure.-,Detoxification,your%20kidneys%20function%20more%20efficiently.)

HORSETAIL

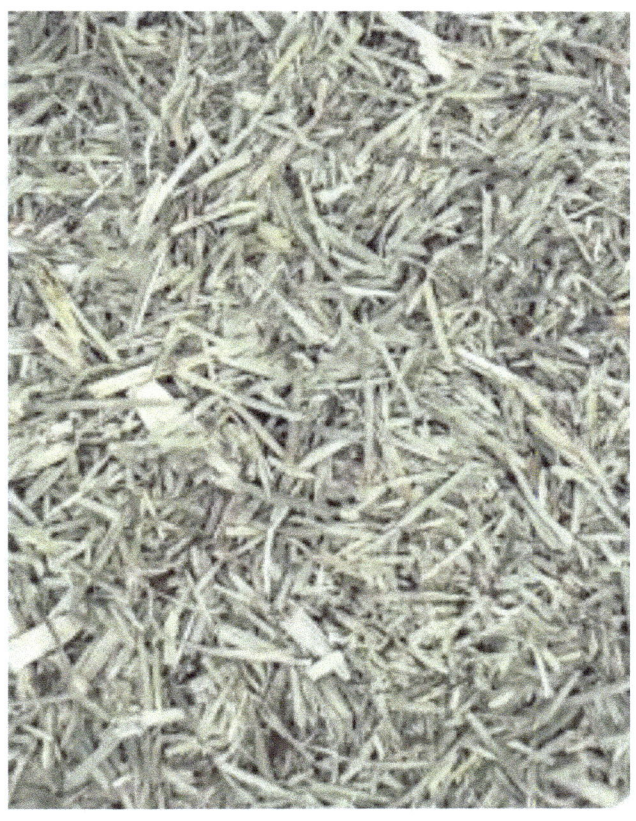

Horsetail is an herbal remedy traditionally used for its many health-promoting effects. Due to its anti-inflammatory and diuretic effects, horsetail can be used to help with treatment of kidney stones and urinary tract infections.
(https://www.tuasaude.com/en/horsetail-tea/)

ROSEMARY

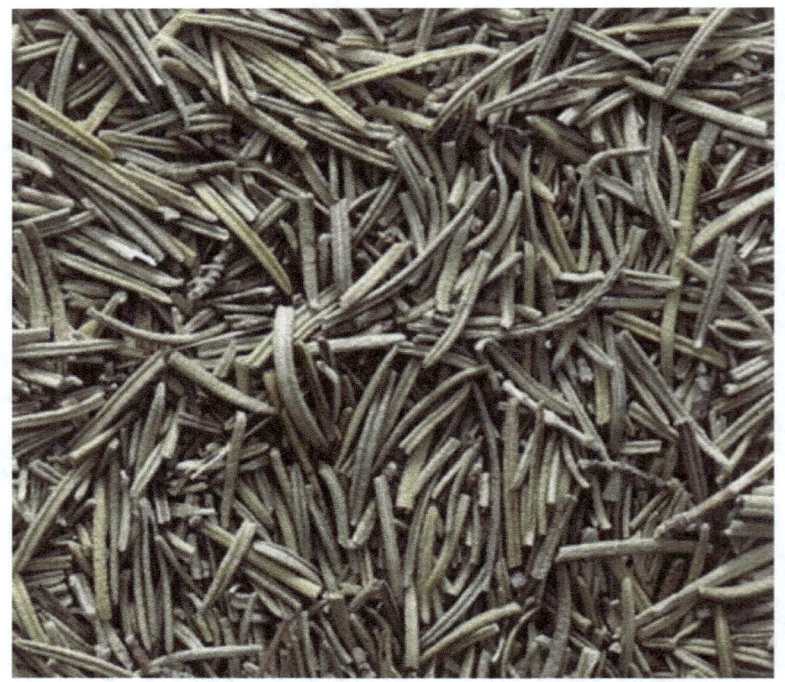

Rosemary - Salvia rosmarinus commonly known as rosemary, is a shrub with fragrant, evergreen, needle-like leaves and white, pink, purple, or blue flowers. Rosemary inhibits the action of the enzyme urease, which helps to form uric acid crystals. Thus, making it a good herbal remedy for preventing and treating kidney stones.
(https://ladyoftheherbs.co.za/2019/03/14/kidney-health-and-5-herbs-to-support-it/)

STINGING NETTLES LEAF

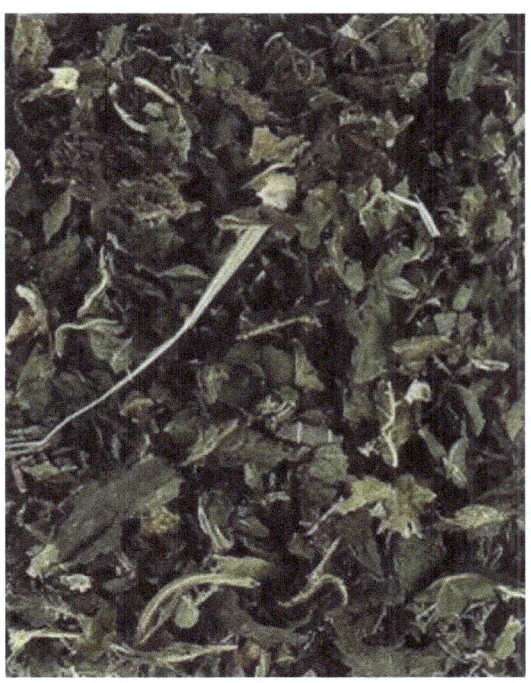

Stinging Nettles leaf is an extract of either the leaves and flowering parts or the roots of Urtica dioica, a tall herbaceous plant found throughout the world in temperate and humid areas. Nettle tea benefits the kidneys by increasing urine output and uric acid removal. Because of its anti-inflammatory properties, it improves kidney function and urinary flow. Nettle tea is a natural diuretic that promotes proper fluid flow in the kidneys and bladder, preventing kidney stones from forming. (https://www.medicinenet.com/what_are_the_benefits_of_drinking_nettle_tea/article.)

GOLDENROD

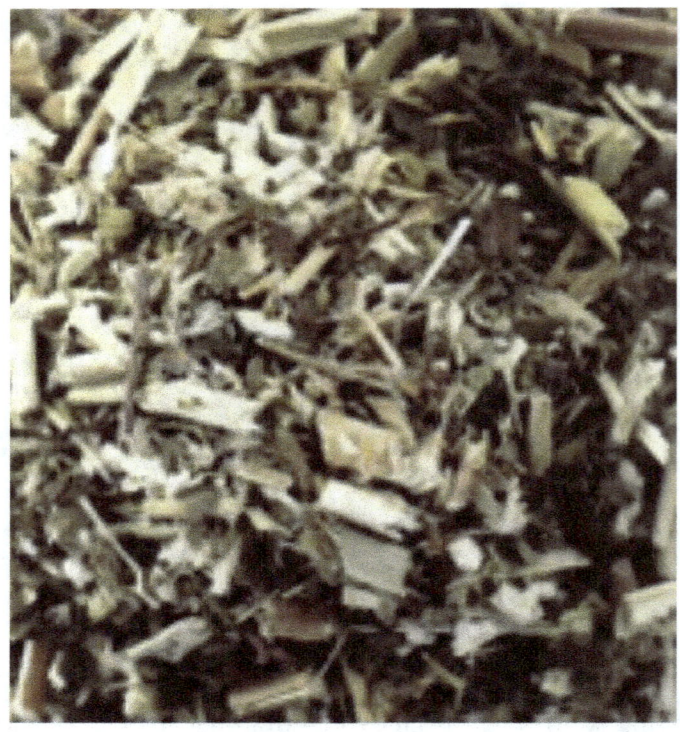

Goldenrod is a common name for many species of flowering plants in the sunflower family, Asteraceae, commonly in reference to the genus Solidago. It seems to act like a diuretic and is used in Europe to treat urinary tract inflammation and to prevent or treat kidney stones. In fact, goldenrod is often found in teas to help "flush out" kidney stones and stop inflammatory diseases of the urinary tract. (https://www.mountsinai.org/health-library/herb/goldenrod #:~:text=It%20does%20seem%20to%20act,often%20blam ed%20for%20seasonal%20allergies)

Chapter 5

Liver

The liver has many functions, including digesting your food and processing and distributing nutrients. There are many kinds of liver disease and conditions. Some, like hepatitis, are caused by viruses. Others can be the result of drugs or drinking too much alcohol. Long-lasting injury or scar tissue in the liver can cause cirrhosis. Jaundice, or yellowing of the skin, can be one sign of liver disease.

This herbal tea blend intake has likewise been shown to protect against various liver conditions, including liver cancer, hepatitis, cirrhosis, fatty liver (hepatic steatosis), and chronic liver disease. Consume 2-3 glasses daily.

Liver Disease Tea

1. Green Tea

2. Ginger Root

3. Dandelion Root

4. Turmeric

5. Milk Thistle

GREEN TEA

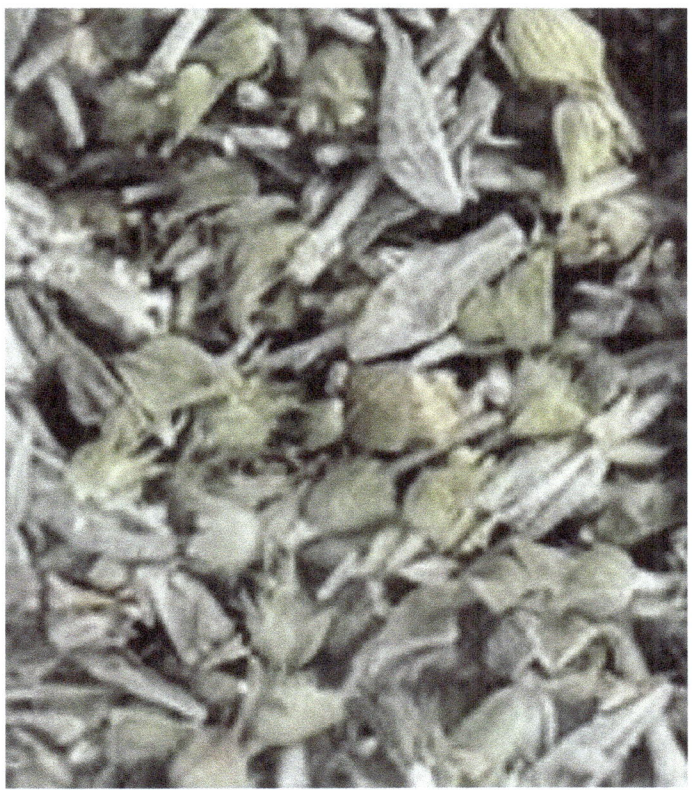

Green Tea is a type of tea that is made from Camellia sinensis leaves and buds that have not undergone the same withering and oxidation process which is used to make oolong teas and black teas. Recent studies have shown that green tea has a certain degree of both preventive and therapeutic effects on liver disease.
(https://www.ncbi.nlm.nih.gov/books/NBK54792)

GINGER ROOT

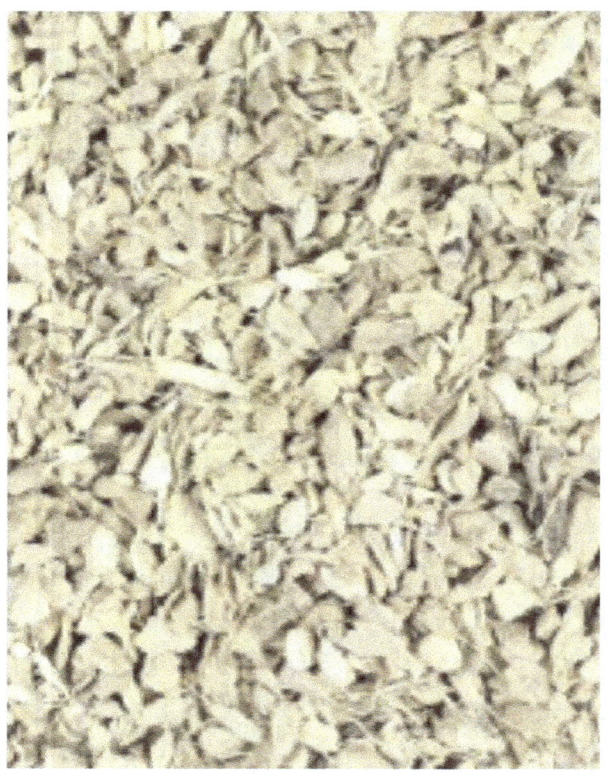

Ginger root contains compounds that may help support liver health, including gingerols and shogaols, which can reduce inflammation and protect cells from damage. Ginger may also help protect the liver from toxins like alcohol.
https://www.ncbi.nlm.nih.gov/pmc/articles/PMC4834197/)

DANDELION ROOT

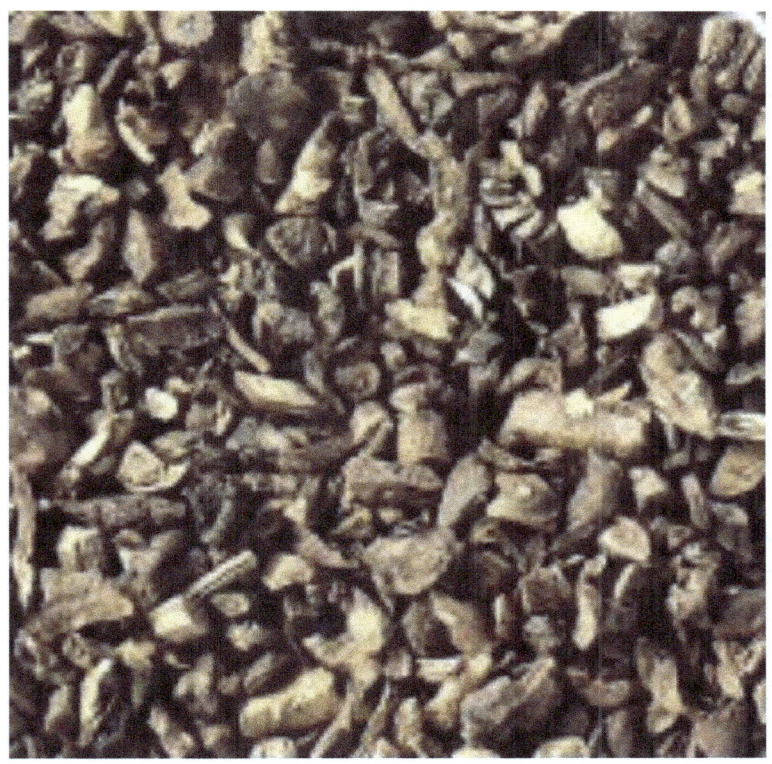

Dandelion root may help detoxify the liver and relieve symptoms of liver disease. (https://www.mountsinai.org/health-library/herb/dandelion#:~:text=The%20root%20of%20the%20dandelion,improve%20liver%20and%20gallbladder%20function.)

TUMERIC

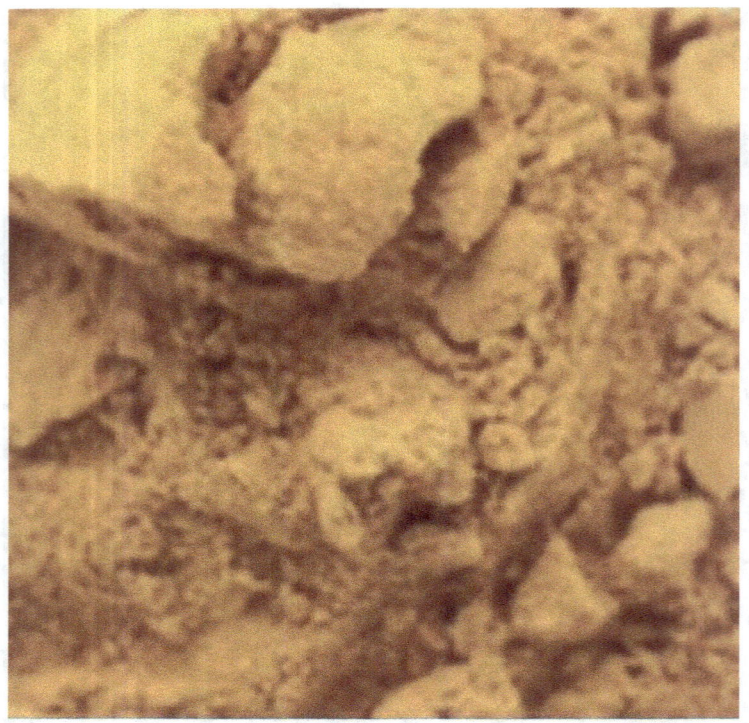

Turmeric - Curcumin is the main ingredient in turmeric, an active ingredient that can eliminate leptin's effects, which is the main cause of cirrhosis. In addition, turmeric also aids bile production, which supports the liver detoxification process and prevents fat build-up in the body while restoring liver function.
(https://www.jeffersonhealth.org/your-health/living-well/the-trouble-with-turmeric-associated-liver-injuries)

MILK THISTLE

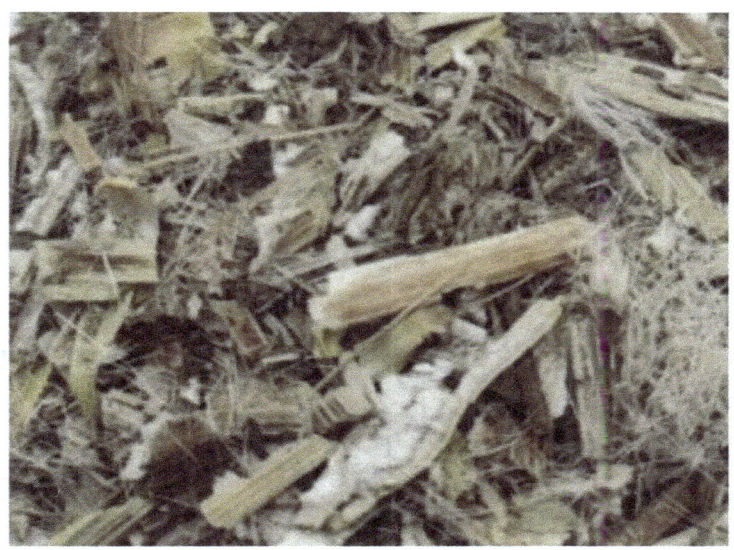

Milk Thistle (silymarin) is a flowering herb related to the daisy and ragweed family. It is native to Mediterranean countries. Several scientific studies suggest that substances in milk thistle (especially a flavonoid called silymarin) protect the liver from toxins, including certain drugs, such as acetaminophen (Tylenol), which can cause liver damage in high doses. Silymarin has antioxidant and anti-inflammatory properties. (https://www.mountsinai.org/health-library/herb/milk-thistle#:~:text=Several%20scientific%20studies%20suggest%20that,antioxidant%20and%20anti%2Dinflammatory%20properties.)

Chapter 6

Brain Disease

Brain Disease can affect how well someone can function and perform daily activities. Some common brain diseases include brain tumors, which can press on nerves and affect brain function, and degenerative nerve diseases, which can affect many of your body's activities, such as balance, movement, talking, breathing, and heart function. The types of brain diseases include Alzheimer's disease and Parkinson's disease.

This herbal blend can help with memory loss. These herbs stimulate the brain. This popular tea blend has been used for centuries to improve cognitive function and enhance memory.

Brain Disease Tea

1. Ginkgo

2. Saffron

3. Turmeric

4. Ashwagandha

5. Lemon Balm

GINGKO

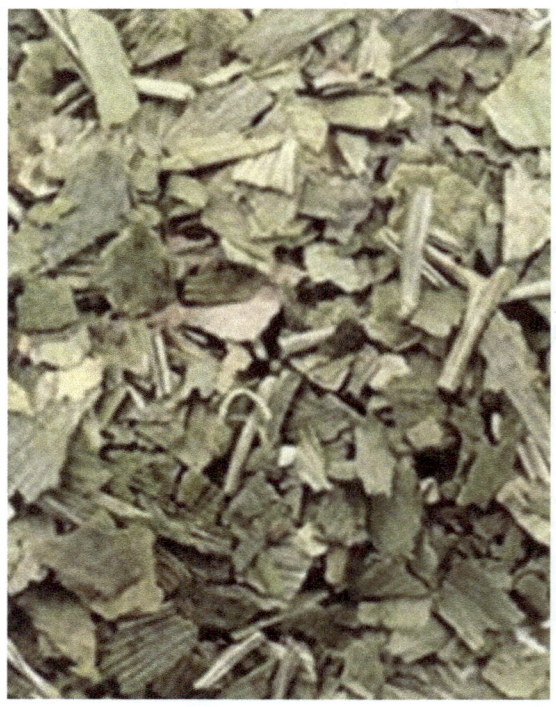

Ginkgo biloba, commonly known as ginkgo or gingko, also known as the maidenhair tree, is a species of gymnosperm tree native to East Asia. Ginkgo improves blood flow to the brain and may help ease a number of circulation problems, including vascular dementia and leg pain caused by clogged arteries.
(https://www.webmd.com/vitamins-and-supplements/supplement-guide-ginkgo-biloba)

SAFFRON

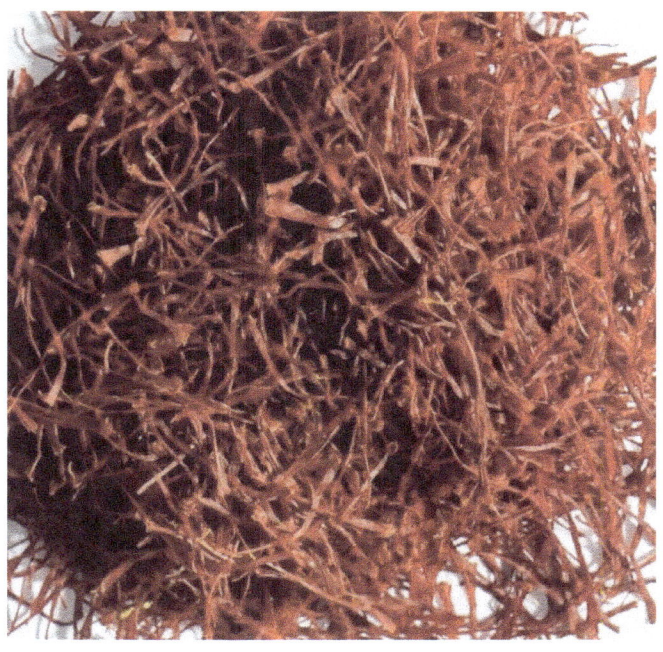

Saffron is a spice derived from the flower of Crocus sativus, commonly known as the "saffron crocus." Saffron and its constituents may have neuroprotective effects that could help with brain health. Saffron contains antioxidants like crocin and crocetin, which may help improve memory function and reduce inflammation and oxidative damage in the brain.

(https://pubmed.ncbi.nlm.nih.gov/38446350/#:~:text=One%20of%20the%20most%20promising,disease%2C%20and%20other%20brain%20disorders.)

TURMERIC

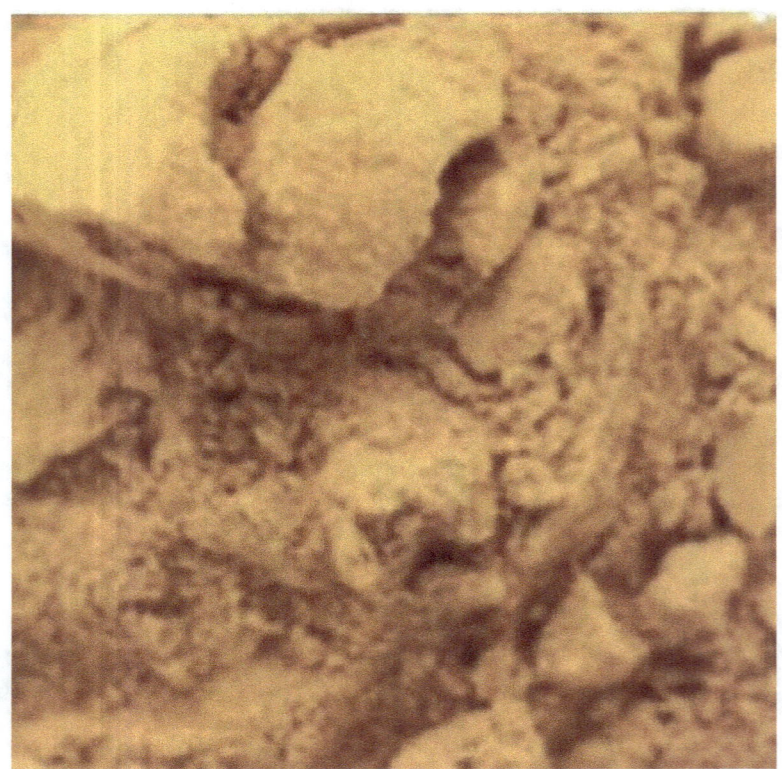

Turmeric and its compound curcumin may have several benefits for brain health. Its positive effects on the brain include boosting the brain neurotransmitters serotonin and dopamine, reducing inflammation, and encouraging brain plasticity.
(https://www.healthline.com/nutrition/top-10-evidence-based-health-benefits-of-turmeric)

ASHWAGANDHA

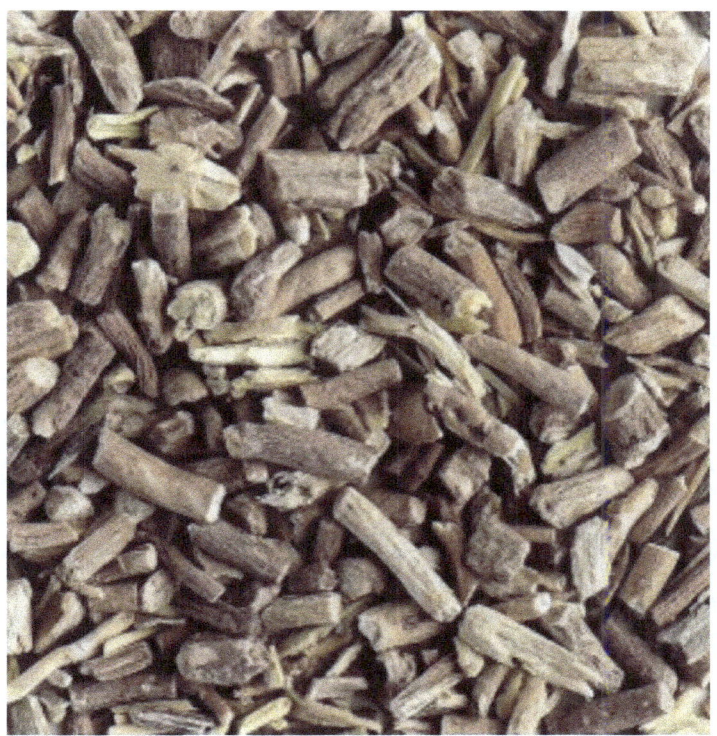

Ashwagandha contains chemicals that might help calm the brain, reduce swelling, lower blood pressure, and alter the immune system. The herb ashwagandha improves brain function and may defend against cognitive decline. (https://www.lifeextension.com/magazine/2021/7/ashwagandha-brain benefits?srsltid=AfmBOopO29SPXvWZHTigtAT UEqTdzs1zJblV5jNq9h-igxoLzeC61eLv)

LEMON BALM

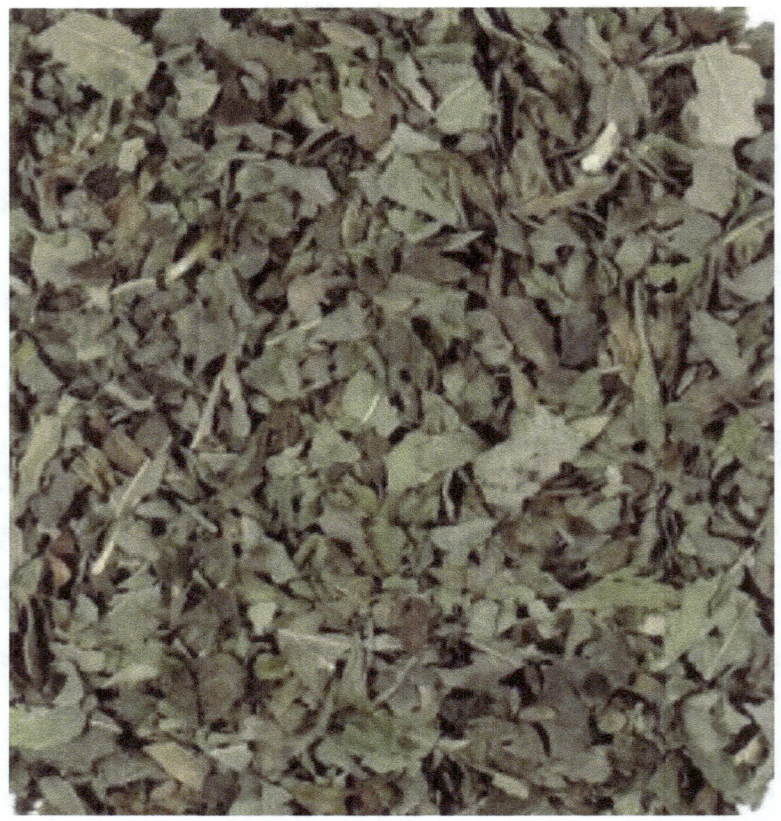

Lemon Balm (Melissa officinalis) is an herb from the mint family. The leaves, which have a mild lemon aroma, are used to make medicine and flavor foods. Lemon Balm undoes damage to the brain caused by chronic stress and oxidative damage. (https://nootropicsexpert.com/lemon-balm/)

Chapter 7

Lung Cancer

Lung cancer is a cancer that begins in the lungs and most often occurs in people who smoke. Two major types of lung cancers are non-small cell lung cancer and small cell lung cancer. Causes of lung cancer include smoking, secondhand smoke, exposure to certain toxins, and family history.

This herbal blend has preventive effects on lung cancer and has a protective effect on lung cancer statistically. The intake of this herbal blend can decrease the lung cancer risk in smoking populations.

Lung Cancer Tea

1. Astragalus Root

2. Lung Wort

3. Echinacea Root

4. Mullein Leaf

5. Sage Leaf

ASTRAGALUS ROOT

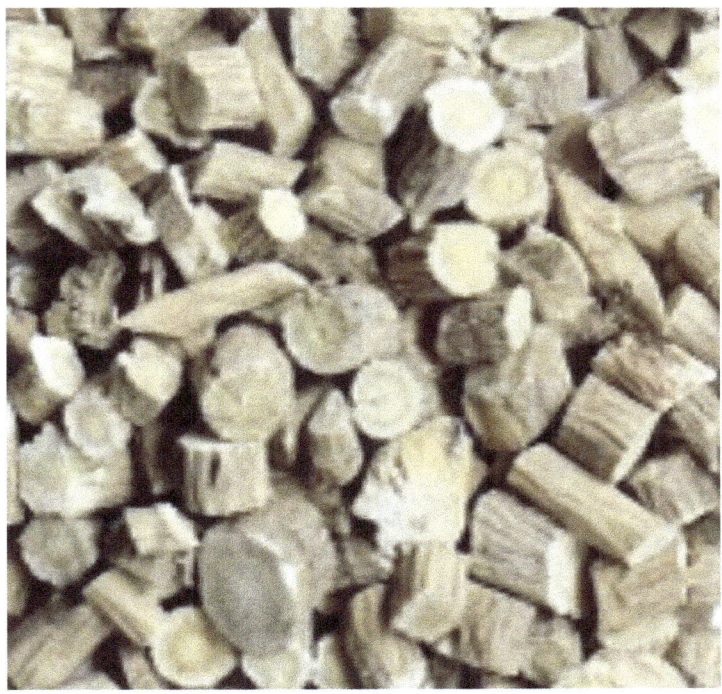

Astragalus root (Astragalus membranaceus) is a type of flowering plant. Astragalus has been used in traditional Chinese medicine for centuries to treat many conditions, including upper respiratory infections and asthma. Some say it can also stimulate the lungs, circulatory system, and urinary system.
(https://www.webmd.com/heart/astragalus-root-heart-benefits-side-effects#:~:text=Proponents%20also%20say%20astragalus%20stimulates,blood%20sugar%20and%20blood%20pressure.)

LUNGWORT

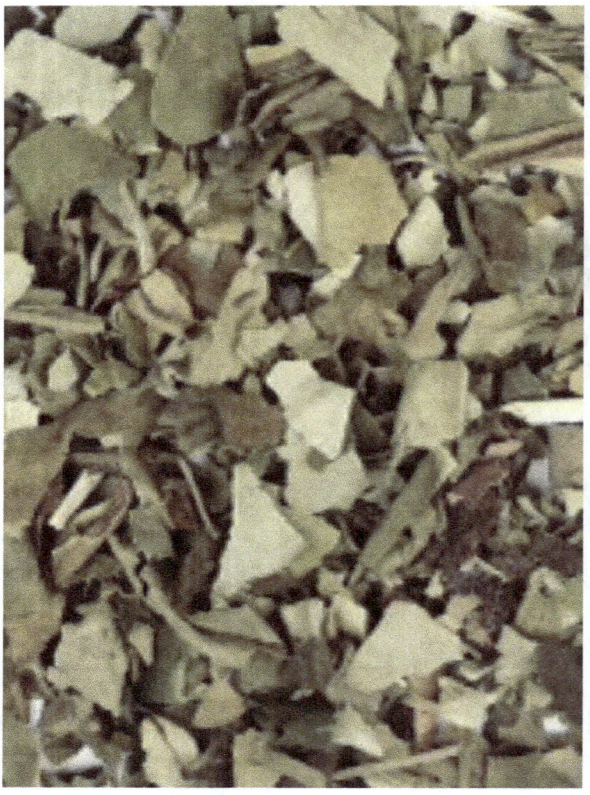

Lungwort Pulmonaria (lungwort) is a genus of flowering plants in the family Boraginaceae, native to Europe and western Asia.

Lungmoss, also called lungwort or lung lichen, is an herbal remedy that's believed to support the lungs and treat breathing conditions. (https://www.healthline.com/health/lungmoss)

ECHINACEA

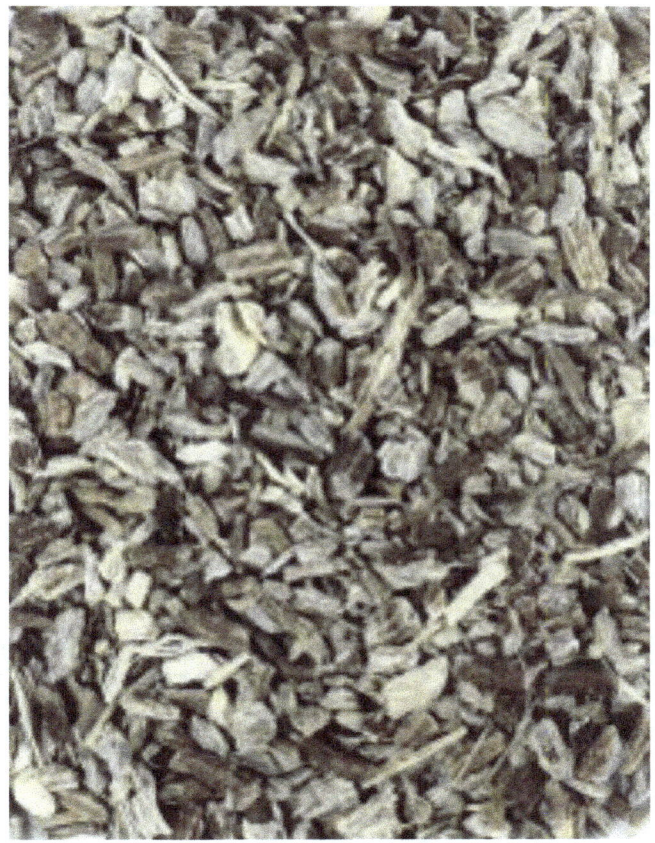

Echinacea root or coneflower is a purple medicinal herb used for common colds, toothaches, and improvement of the overall immune system. Echinacea is an herb widely used for the prevention or treatment of upper respiratory tract infections.
(https://pubmed.ncbi.nlm.nih.gov/15813158/)

MULLEIN LEAF

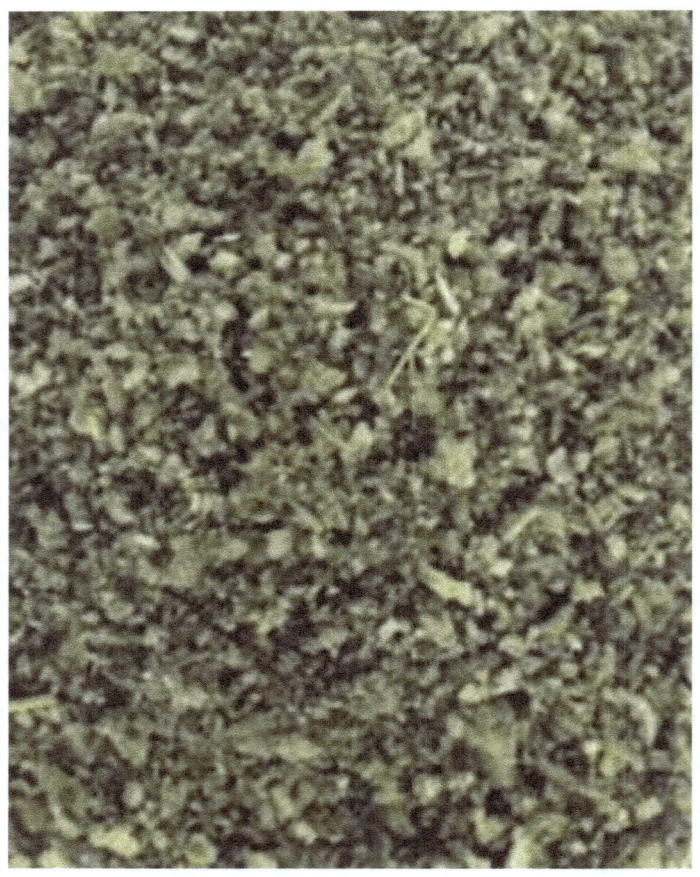

Mullein leaf (Verbascum densiflorum) is a flowering plant found in mountain areas. Mullein leaf is well known for its positive effect on the respiratory system as well as the lungs. (https://www.webmd.com/vitamins/ai/ingredientmono-572/mullein)

SAGE LEAF

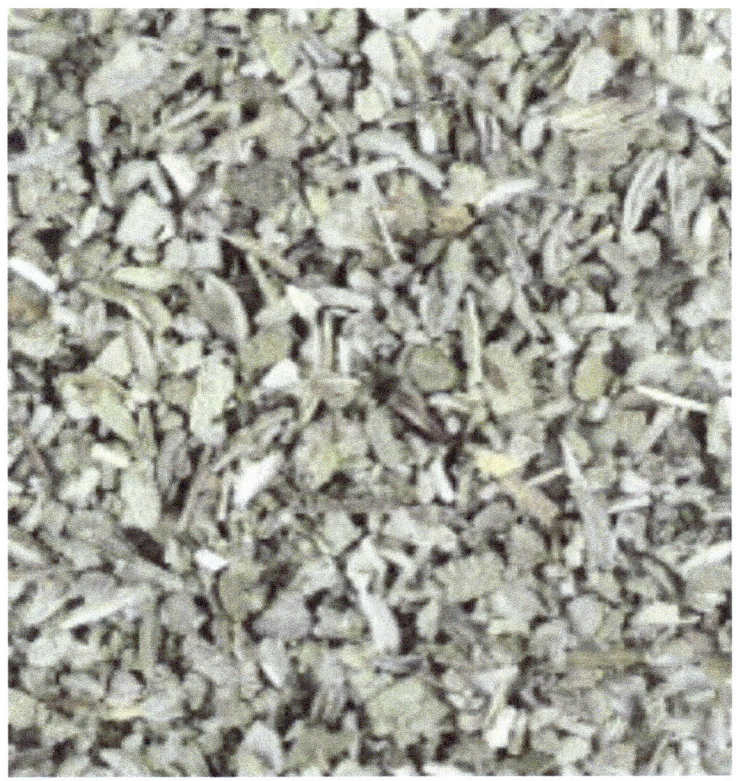

Sage leaf has anti-inflammatory, antioxidant, and antimicrobial properties. Sage tea can help with respiratory problems and is useful in treating lung disorders.
(https://ancientfoods.com/blogs/journal/sage-tea-is-beneficial-for-lung-health#:~:text=Salvia%20offic inalis%20has%20antibacterial%2C%20astringent, usefulness%20in%20treating%20lung%20disorder s.%22)

Chapter 8

Diabetes (Diabetes Mellitus)

Diabetes can result in too much sugar in the blood. (High Blood Glucose) There are four types of diabetes.

1. Gestational diabetes is a condition that causes high blood sugar during pregnancy.

2. Prediabetes is a blood sugar level that is higher than what's considered healthy but not high enough to be type 2 diabetes.

3. Type 1 diabetes is a lifelong condition where the pancreas makes little or no insulin, which leads to high blood sugar levels.

4. Type 2 diabetes is a long-term condition in which the body has trouble controlling blood sugar and using it for energy.

This herbal blend helps lower blood sugar in people with diabetes. It also increases lean body mass, improves muscle strength and endurance, and accelerates the rate of glycogen resynthesis during post-exercise recovery. Consume 2-3 glasses daily.

Diabetes Tea

1. Fenugreek

2. Milk Thistle

3. Turmeric

4. Cinnamon

5. Holy Basil

FENUGREEK

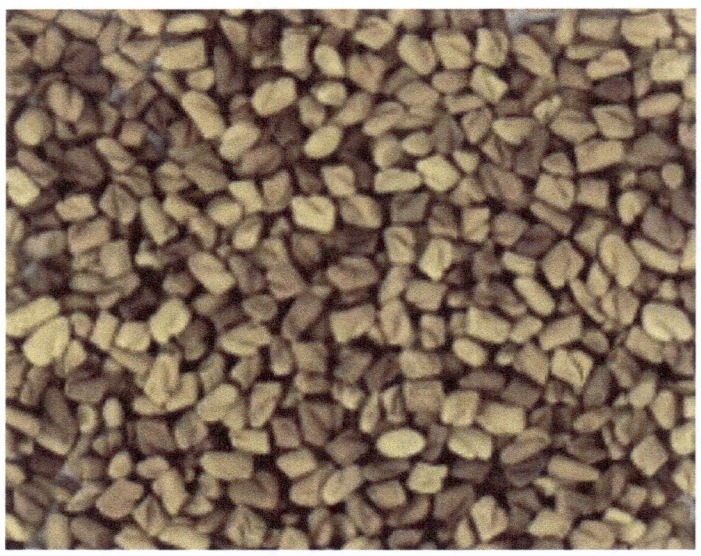

Fenugreek (Trigonella foenum-graecum) is an herb similar to clover. The seeds taste similar to maple syrup and are used in foods and medicine. Fenugreek seeds (Trigonella foenumgraecum) have been used in traditional medicine as a complementary therapy for diabetes. Research suggests that fenugreek may have antidiabetic properties that can help manage diabetes by lowering blood sugar, improving insulin sensitivity, delaying gastric emptying, and reducing glucose absorption. (https://www.medicalnewstoday.com/articles/can-fenugreek-help-manage-diabetes.)

MILK THISTLE

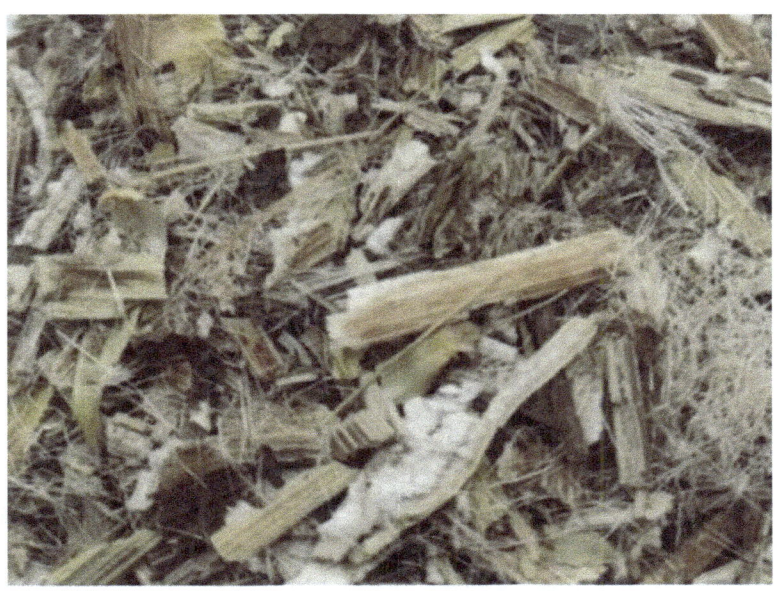

Milk Thistle - Medical research suggests that milk thistle, combined with traditional treatment, can improve diabetes.

(https://www.webmd.com/digestive-disorders/milk-thistle-benefits-and-side-effects)

TURMERIC

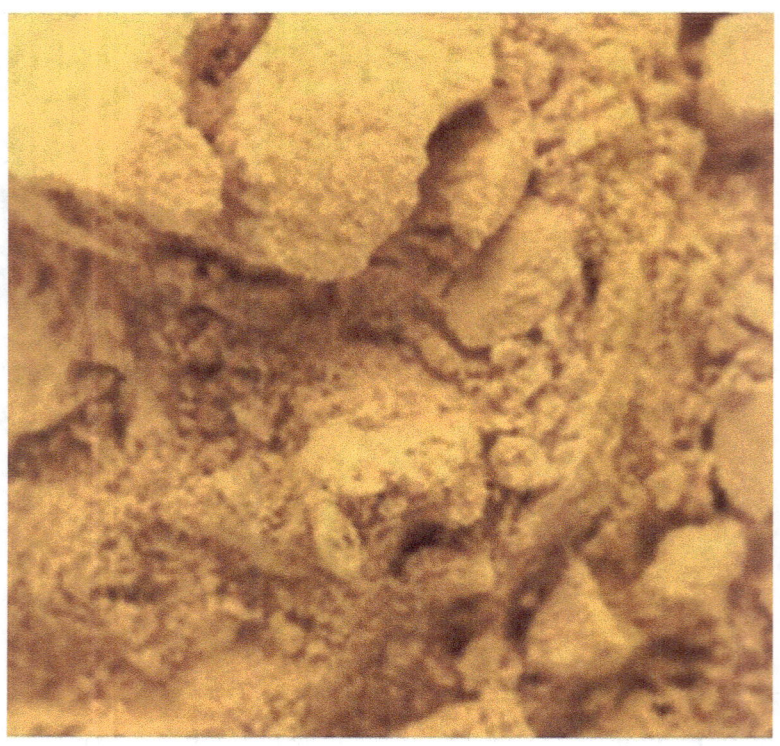

Turmeric's active component, curcumin can decrease blood sugar levels and reduce diabetes-related complications. Curcumin may also have a role in diabetes prevention.
(https://www.healthline.com/health

CINNAMON

Cinnamon - Research has suggested that cinnamon can help to improve blood glucose levels and increase insulin sensitivity. (https://www.diabetes.co.uk/natural-therapies/cinnamon.html)

HOLY BASIL

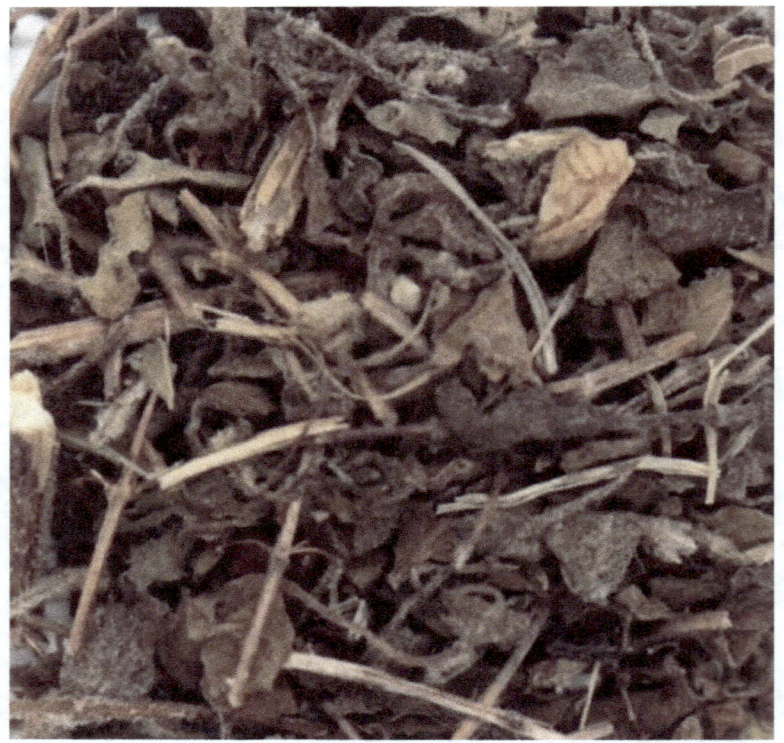

Holy basil - If you have prediabetes or type 2 diabetes, all parts of the holy basil plant can help reduce your blood sugar. Holy basil can help prevent symptoms of diabetes such as: weight gain. hyperinsulinemia, or excess insulin in the blood.
(https://www.healthline.com/health/food-nutrition/basil-benefits#:~:text=If%20you%20have%20prediabetes%20or,excess%20insulin%20in%20the%20blood)

Chapter 9

Prostate Cancer

Prostate Cancer is in a man's prostate, a small walnut-sized gland that produces seminal fluid. A man's prostate produces the seminal fluid that nourishes and transports sperm. Some types of prostate cancer grow slowly. In some cases, monitoring is recommended, and other types of prostate cancer can be very aggressive.

This herbal tea blend helps kill cancer cells while keeping healthy cells intact. Cancer cells divide more frequently than most normal cells, and different cells fight different types of cancer. Consume 2-3 glasses daily.

Prostate Cancer Tea

1. Ginger Root

2. Turmeric

3. Sour sop leaves

4. St. John's Wort

GINGER ROOT

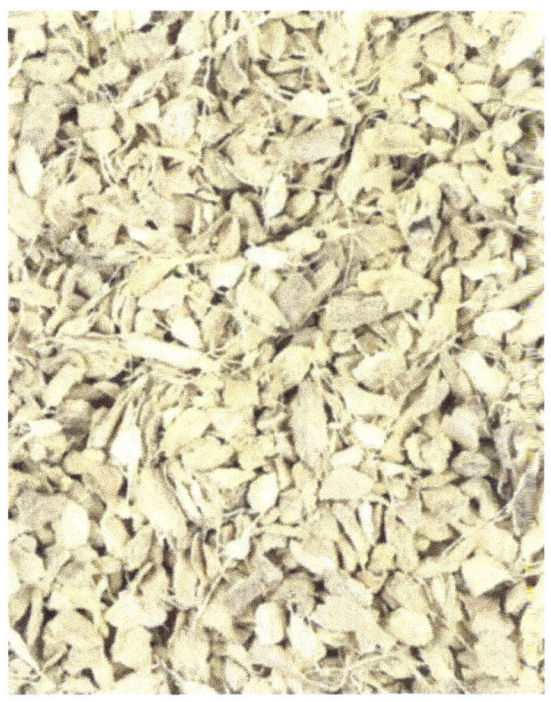

Ginger root contains vitamins A, C and E, beta-carotene and zinc, all strong antioxidants that protect the prostate from harmful free radicals. Free radicals speed up tissue aging and cancer development.

(https://urologyexperts.com/ginger-can-help-fight-prostatecancer/.)

TURMERIC

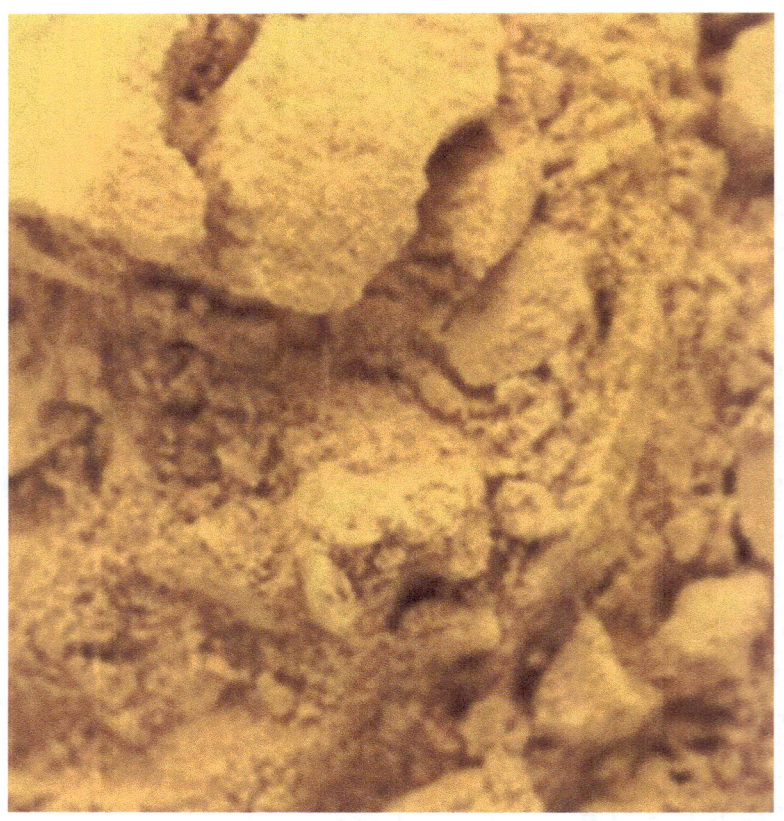

Turmeric - Researchers have found that turmeric and its extract, curcumin, may help prevent or treat prostate cancer. (**https://www.healthline.com/health/prosta te-cancer/turmeric-and-prostate-cancer**)

SOURSOP LEAVES

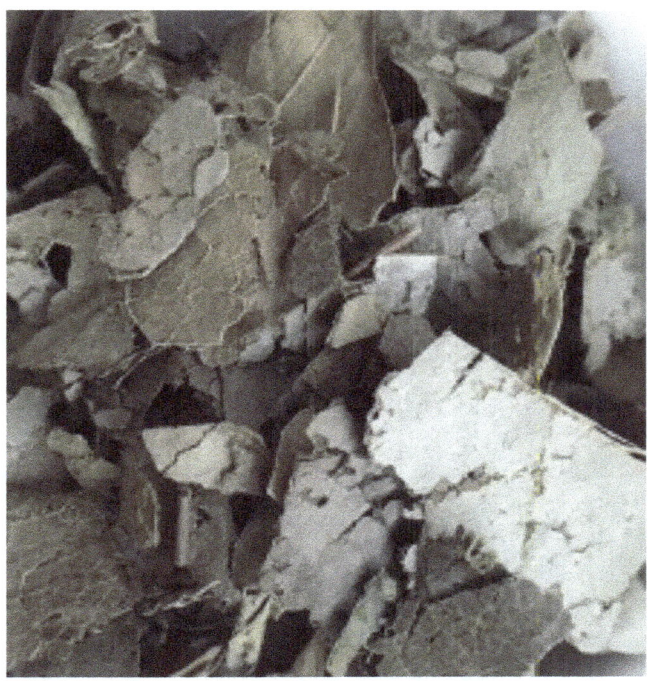

Soursop leaves known as guanabana or graviola is an exotic fruit known for having a high content of vitamin C and antioxidants. Soursop, also known as Brazilian paw paw, has been used in traditional healing for its leaves, fruit, and bark. Some studies have shown that soursop's active ingredients may have potential benefits for the prostate, including inhibiting tumor growth and reducing prostate size. (https://www.cancerresearchuk.org/about-cancer/treatment/complementary-alternative-therapies/individual-therapies/graviola)

ST JOHN'S WORT

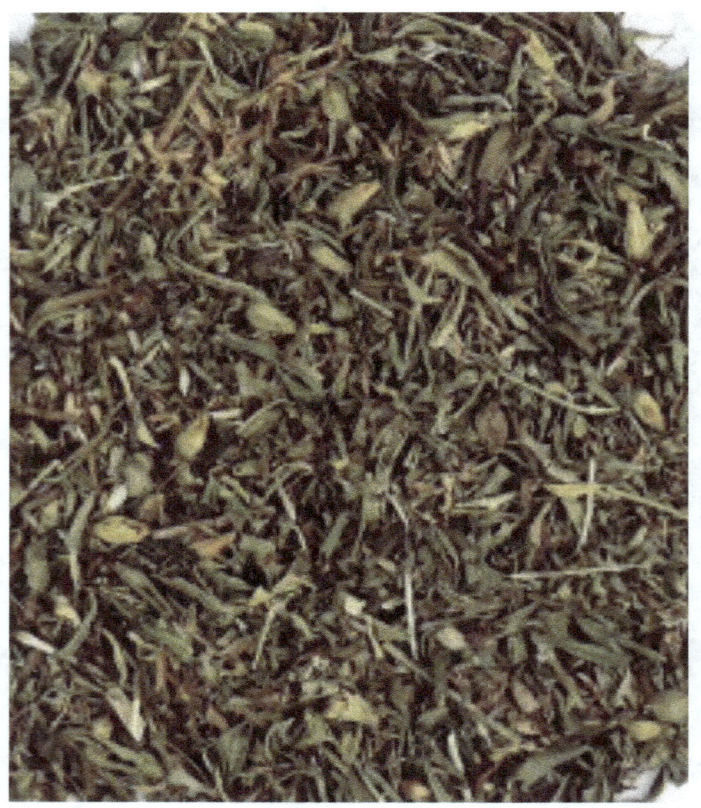

St. John's wort is a plant with yellow flowers that has been used in traditional European medicine as far back as the ancient Greeks. St. John's wort has antibacterial, antioxidant, anti-inflammatory, and antiviral properties.
(https://www.mountsinai.org/health-library/herb/st-johns-wort)

This book is a simple guide that explores the powerful impact of herbal teas in managing and improving your health. By harnessing the natural properties of various herbs, this book offers remedies for a wide range of ailments, from digestive issues to chronic illnesses. It emphasizes the importance of discipline in diet and the healing process, encouraging readers to trust the natural detoxification power of these herbal concoctions.

Learn how the right combinations of teas can help flush out harmful toxins, including mucus, cancers, parasites, and metal calcifications, promoting overall wellness. Alongside these teas, this book also highlights the importance of hydration and proper fluid intake to support your body's cleansing processes. Trust in nature, trust in the process, and embark on a journey towards a healthier, toxin-free life.

About the Author - ChrisAngela Spencer

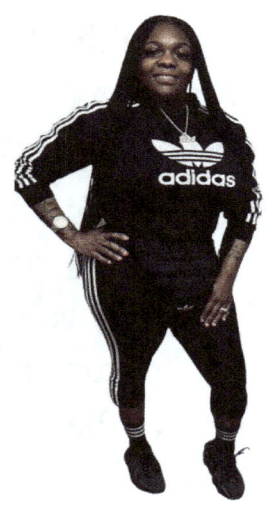

ChrisAngela Spencer is a mother of seven from Atlanta, Georgia. She is a teacher with 13 years of teaching experience. Her professional development is a critical part of growth that can directly impact students' ability to learn. ChrisAngela has her Child Development Associate (CDA) and also her Technical Certificate of Credit (TCC). Teaching is her passion, and she loves to promote the importance of education. She wrote this book for people with certain diseases to help cure themselves using different herbs from nature.

www.ingramcontent.com/pod-product-compliance
Lightning Source LLC
Chambersburg PA
CBHW070317290526
45791CB00003B/1152